Complete Method For Managing Reflux Symptoms

Malia Kōnane

Published by Editorial Atelerix Creative Quill, 2022.

COMPLETE METHOD FOR MANAGING REFLUX SYMPTOMS

First edition. April 30, 2022.

ISBN: 979-8215159293

Written by Malia Kōnane.

Also by Malia Kōnane

Ultimate Leading Guide for Women
Extreme Rapid Weight Loss For Woman
The Struggle With Weight Loss and Weight Gain and Overcoming
Obstacles
Awakening From Consciousness
Be Your Own Excellence
False Identity
How To Compose The Perfect Song For Yourself
The Power Of Knowing You: "Conquer Your Life And Be Happy."
You will Wish to be Born Again
Anger Management for Parents
Complete Method For Managing Reflux Symptoms
False Identity Volume 2 The Mental Hell Of The Narcissist
Food Blog Definitive Guide
Gastric Band Hypnosis for Women Stop Emotional Eating & Sugar
Cravings and Achieve Extreme Rapid Weight Loss
Handuka Strategy The Five O's.
Human Future: What Will our Stamp in Time be?
Mindfulness And Mental Health Well-Being
Mobile Homes: The Housing Problem Solution Of Xxi Century
Motherhood and Moneymaking: Crush Those Goals, Make That
Money, Raise Those Kids
Own Your Vibration
Resilience: Mastering The Art of Taking Whatever Sh*t Life Throws At
You

Word Of Lies

Table of Contents

To my family and friends who always support me.

I am a freelance author with a very tight budget to publish books, but I do it with a lot of love and affection; I would appreciate a review from you to help me maintain my love of literature and writing.

Thank you from all my heart.

Malia Kōnane

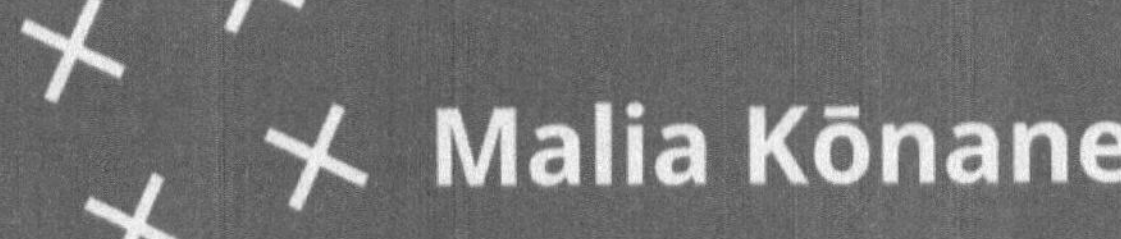

Complete Method for Managing Reflux Symptoms

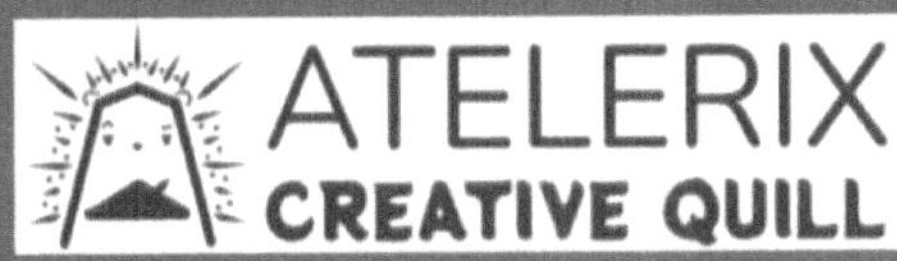

Complete Method For Managing Reflux Symptoms

REFLUX STRIKES AGAIN

An Underestimated Disease

Gastroesophageal reflux occurs when stomach contents back up into the esophagus. Gastric acid that touches the lining of the esophagus can cause heartburn, also known as acid indigestion. Doctors also refer to gastroesophageal reflux as:

- Acid indigestion
- Gastric reflux
- Regurgitation
- Heartburn
- Reflux
- Acid reflux

Gastroesophageal reflux is a common problem that occurs when acid from the stomach frequently flows into the tube that connects the mouth and stomach's esophagus. Acid reflux can irritate the lining of the esophagus. In the passage of stomach contents into the esophagus, between the esophagus and the stomach, there is a natural barrier formed by the lower esophageal sphincter that opens to allow the passage of ingested material into the stomach and, at the same time, prevents the natural passage gastric contents into the esophagus, when this mechanism fails frequently or continuously is when this condition occurs.

This barrier mechanism fails when the pressure of the lower esophageal sphincter is

permanently low or more frequently when the relaxation of this sphincter occurs at a time when there is no progression of ingested material through the esophagus. When this happens, all the acidic contents of the stomach irritate or injure the esophageal mucosa that is not prepared to support acidic materials like the stomach is.

Many people have acid reflux periodically. Gastroesophageal reflux disease can be defined as mild acid reflux that happens at least twice a week or more severe acid reflux that occurs at least once a week. It is very common to have acid reflux occasionally, and, in fact, almost everyone feels it sometimes. Still, acid reflux becomes a problem when it occurs often, involves a lot of acids, or affects the part of the esophagus closest to the throat.

Almost everyone has at some moments transitory passage of gastric content to the esophagus caused by some circumstance. Still, it is only considered a disease when this produces symptoms. These are frequent and/or intense enough to deteriorate the quality of life of the person.

Conditions that cause acid reflux

A hiatal hernia (part of the stomach displaced into the thoracic cavity through the diaphragmatic hiatus) facilitates the presence of reflux. However, there are many people who have acid reflux without a hiatal hernia.

Anything that increases intra-abdominal pressure also promotes acid reflux. This is the case of pregnancy, ventral (forward) flexion positions of the trunk, or very tight dresses or belts. The decubitus position (lying down) also favors it by a simple matter of gravity.

Obesity, or an increase in abdominal girth, favors reflux. However, sometimes only moderate increases in weight or this perimeter can trigger or aggravate it.

Diagnosis of reflux

The most characteristic symptoms are a burning sensation (called heartburn) that begins in the upper and central part of the abdomen and moves up to the chest and neck. The consequent regurgitation of fluid into the mouth, especially when you are lying on the bed. It generally worsens after meals, especially with foods that promote sphincter relaxation or dietary excesses. In a lot of cases, it also worsens during night rest or when the trunk is flexed.

Other digestive symptoms can be discomfort or pain when swallowing food or liquids, frequent belching, or sore throat.

Gastroesophageal reflux disease can also present non-digestive symptoms, such as angina-like chest pain, chronic cough, chronic pharyngitis, or bronchial asthma.

In the absence of troublesome symptoms such as anemia, difficulty swallowing, or unnecessary weight loss, the continued and frequent presence of heartburn and/or regurgitation can be considered a diagnosis of reflux without the need for specific tests.

In the case of evaluating the severity of the disease or knowing if there are obvious lesions of the esophageal mucosa, and upper digestive endoscopy must be performed. This test consists of the introduction of a tube through the mouth through which we can see the interior of the esophagus and the stomach. The examination is not painful, but it is a bit uncomfortable because it causes nausea. However, it is done quickly (around 5-10 minutes), which minimizes discomfort.

In some specific and rare cases of diagnostic doubts or poor treatment progress, another examination must be performed. The acid content of the esophagus is measured using a pH probe (24-hour pH-metry).

Not all reflux manifests in the same way

Types of reflux

Gastroesophageal reflux consists of the retrograde passage of gastric contents to the esophagus. Classically, this concept has been assimilated to the passage of acid content since it was only possible to measure it by pH-metry, which does not allow the detection of reflux episodes that do not produce a decrease in intraesophageal pH. The subsequent availability of other techniques, such as Bilitec® and, more recently, the measurement of intraesophageal impedance, has allowed the recording of non-acid gastroesophageal reflux episodes. The classification takes into account the degree of acidity of the refluxed material (acid reflux/ weak acid, reflux/non-acid reflux), the reflux chemical composition (bile reflux), and its physical state (liquid reflux/gas reflux).

Non-acid reflux

Previously, this term has often been used to refer to episodes of reflux that do not cause a decrease in esophageal pH, for those that produce decreases in pH that do not reach the value of 4, for those that produce decreases in pH slighter than a period, and even for bile reflux. At present, it has been agreed that there are episodes of gastroesophageal reflux that do not cause a decrease in esophageal pH below 7. Therefore, it has been said that this term should be replaced by "weak alkaline reflux."

In cases where the reflux episode, detected by impedance measurement, occurs when the esophageal pH is lower than 7, and there are no changes in said pH, the term "weak acid reflux" should be applied. This situation is especially common in neonates, in whom gastric pH is usually higher than esophageal. Its registration is only possible through the simultaneous use of pH-metry and impedance measurement.

Weakly acid reflux

Weakly acid reflux refers to episodes of gastroesophageal reflux that cause a decrease in esophageal pH to values between 4 and 7. Not considering these episodes implies an underestimation of gastroesophageal reflux, especially in the postprandial period, when gastric pH is usually at values higher than 4.

This circumstance is especially important in children, especially in infants, given the high frequency of their ingestions. In them, it has been estimated that more than two-thirds of reflux episodes do not cause a decrease in esophageal pH below 4. Although this type of gastroesophageal reflux can be detected by esophageal pH-metry, analyzing drops in pH greater than one point, even when they do not reach the pH of 4, the combined use of pH-metry and impedance measurement improves their detection.

Acid reflux

It has been agreed to consider it when the intraesophageal pH falls below 4, caused by the retrograde passage of gastric content (therefore, in the absence of ingestion of acidic material). Its measurement has been carried out classically by means of pH-metry, although different technical aspects question its reliability. Among others, the standardization of the reading of the record, the swallowing of acidic material, and the changes in the position of the pH probe with respect to the esophagus can make it difficult to interpret the record properly. On the other hand, the simultaneous measurement of pH and esophageal impedance offers a significant improvement for the interpretation of doubtful situations.

Reflux episodes that occur when the esophageal pH is already below 4 deserve special comment. In these cases, referred to as "superimposed acid reflux," pH-metry is usually inadequate for its detection since it is often changing in pH, changes do not occur, or such changes are minimal. Also, in this situation, the simultaneous measurement of esophageal pH and impedance is the best solution.

Bile reflux

It consists of the reflux of duodenal contents to the esophagus, marked by the detection of bilirubin. It is also called duodenum-gastric-esophageal reflux or bilirubin reflux. It can accompany both acid and weakly acidic or weakly alkaline reflux.

Gas reflux

The introduction of the esophageal impedance measurement allows distinguishing the physical state of the reflux material, liquid or gaseous. Fluid reflux is recorded as a retrograde decrease in impedance in at least 3 recording points in the distal esophagus. Gas reflux is defined by a simultaneous or retrograde increase in impedance in two esophageal segments, independent of swallowing.

In patients with reflux disease rather than sporadic reflux, mixed gas and liquid reflux are more common than exclusively liquid reflux. In these cases of mixed reflux, either one can precede the other.

GER vs. GERD

Acid reflux (GER) occurs when stomach acid backs up into the esophagus, or tube that connects the throat to the stomach. When there is acid reflux, the person may have a taste of sour food or liquid at the end of the mouth, pain or pressure in the chest, or a burning sensation in the chest, known as heartburn.

When the acid reflux leads to frequent symptoms or complications, then it is renamed gastroesophageal reflux disease or GERD, a condition that often requires treatment. If you have reflux symptoms more than twice a month, see your doctor to assess the problem. This disease occurs when the valve in the lower part of the esophagus (where it connects to the stomach) becomes weak or relaxes when it should not relax.

GERD is a stronger type of acid reflux. The most seen symptom of GERD is frequent heartburn. However, other signs and symptoms may include spitting up sour food or liquid, difficulty swallowing, coughing, wheezing, and chest pain, especially when lying down at night.

Gastroesophageal reflux disease (GERD) is common. It affects a percentage of between 10 and 20% of adults. It also frequently occurs in children and sometimes begins at birth.

Is it reflux or something else?

You finish dinner, and you feel a strange burning, that feeling that reminds you that you are no longer so young ... or at least not so resistant to some foods and bad habits. But do you know exactly what your discomfort is about? Know the differences between gastritis and reflux; not all burning is the same.

It is essential to know the differences between gastroesophageal reflux and gastritis. It is estimated that about 40% of patients are diagnosed with gastritis and may only have reflux.

Gastroesophageal reflux consists of the rise of gastric content, made up of hydrochloric acid, pepsin, and bile salts, into the esophagus. This content causes discomfort and damage to the esophagus. On the other hand, gastritis is an inflammation of the stomach lining. It is due to a weakness or injury to the mucous barrier that protects the stomach and allows the passage of digestive juices that irritate it. Both diseases are different. However, they share things in common, such as some symptoms and treatment, which may be why we get confused.

Unlike gastritis, which appears as a burning in the "pit of the stomach," with reflux, it occurs in the chest, in addition to feeling a lump in the throat, difficulty swallowing, or sour regurgitation. Other symptoms of gastritis are: pain, burning or a feeling of indigestion in the upper abdomen, feeling full, nausea, and even vomiting. Commonly, everything improves when you eat, but sometimes even that can't help.

Reflux symptoms are common during pregnancy. But they rarely cause complications, such as inflammation of the esophagus (esophagitis). Most of the time, heartburn symptoms improve after the baby is born.

Fortunately, most gastritis is not serious and improves with treatment. However, it is very important to consult your doctor, especially if you have been like this for more than a week. In severe cases, it can cause ulcers and increase the risk of stomach cancer.

UNDERSTANDING YOUR BODY

Main causes of reflux

One of the most important and well-known causes of GERD is the alteration at the level of the lower esophageal sphincter. The latter is a muscular ring that surrounds the esophagus at its junction with the stomach. It remains closed, preventing the contents from the stomach back to the esophagus.

When the sphincter is altered, and there is a decrease in its pressure at rest, it relaxes and does not perform its function well so that the stomach contents reflux. In addition, certain drugs and substances such as alcohol, chocolate, or tobacco favor the relaxation of the sphincter and, therefore, the appearance of reflux.

Another factor that determines the appearance of acid reflux is the alteration of the "esophageal clearance," that is, the ability of the esophagus to quickly and completely empty the refluxed gastric contents.

Finally, the alteration of the resistance of the mucosa to withstand aggressive factors can also favor the onset of this disease and lesions in the esophagus.

On the other hand, some pathologies or situations can increase the chances of suffering from gastroesophageal reflux; then, we will talk about the most common ones.

Obesity

Gastroesophageal reflux and gastroesophageal reflux disease are closely related to obesity; up to 45% of severely obese patients (BMI> 40) suffer from it. Due to the increment in the prevalence of obesity globally, the impact on the etiology and treatment of reflux has become an important point. There are many studies that report the association of reflux with an increase in body mass index.

Different factors produce an increase in the pressure gradient of a gastroesophageal junction seen in obesity, including:

- Increased intra-abdominal pressure.

- Increased intragastric pressure and intrathoracic inspiratory negative pressure.

- The diaphragmatic crura provide the mechanical separation between the LES and the extrinsic compression.

- The latter is essential for the formation of Hiatal hernias, which, according to endoscopic evidence, are more frequent in obese subjects than in normal subjects.

In summary, obesity is the main risk factor for acid reflux and gastroesophageal reflux disease, diseases that a high percentage of the world's population suffers from. Obesity potentiates reflux and inflammation-induced esophageal injury. In addition, excess abdominal fat in the body increases intra-abdominal pressure. This barrier exists between the stomach and the esophagus decreases, which facilitates the rise of gastric acids.

Pregnancy

The majority of pregnant women have symptoms of acid reflux, especially heartburn, at some point. These symptoms can start at any time during pregnancy. And they often get worse throughout pregnancy. For example, heartburn is common when you are pregnant.

The causes of acid reflux during pregnancy are still controversial and have been little studied. However, the most important factors that influence its appearance are the increase in abdominal volume and hormonal factors, which produce a decrease in the pressure of the lower esophageal sphincter.

Even so, in a generalized way, it is considered that heartburn during pregnancy is due to hormones that make the digestive system work more slowly. The muscles in our bodies that push food down the esophagus can also move slower when a woman is pregnant. And as the uterus grows, it increments pressure on the stomach. This can sometimes force stomach acid into the esophagus.

Acid reflux symptoms are common during the pregnancy stage. But they rarely cause complications, such as inflammation of the esophagus (esophagitis). Most of the time, heartburn symptoms improve after the baby is born.

Hiatal hernia

A hiatal hernia is a common anatomical entity affecting 20% of the population. It occurs when the highest part of the stomach protrudes through the large muscle separating the abdomen chest (diaphragm).

The diaphragm of our body has a small opening called hiatus through which the feeding tube (esophagus) passes before joining the stomach. In a hiatal hernia, the stomach pushes up to pass through this hole and into the chest.

90% of Hiatal hernias are by sliding, and in them, the union of the esophagus with the stomach is completely displaced through the hiatus. 5% are para esophageal, in which the junction of the esophagus with the stomach remains in its abdominal position, and it is only the stomach that herniates. The remaining 5% are mixed, a combination of the above.

The predisposing factors to suffer from HH, in addition to the genetic ones, are those that can generate a progressive weakening of the diaphragmatic pillars (or retaining walls) of the hiatus and are: obesity, aging, chronic cough, constipation, stress, smoking, and carrying out very heavy efforts or tasks.

When the hiatal hernia is small, it does not usually cause problems. You may never find out you have one unless your doctor discovers it while checking for another condition.

However, a bigger hiatal hernia can allow food and acid to back up into the esophagus, leading to heartburn. Generally, self-care measures or medications can alleviate these symptoms. However, when the hiatal hernia is very large, it may require surgery.

Connective tissue disorders (scleroderma)

Progressive systemic sclerosis and other degenerative connective tissue diseases often affect the esophagus. For example, in the case of scleroderma, up to 75% of patients with cutaneous manifestations may show esophageal alterations.

Histologically, muscle atrophy and fibrosis are observed, mainly affecting the smooth muscle region of the esophagus. As a result, severe hypomotility is observed, with failure to contract the distal esophagus and hypotonia of the lower esophageal sphincter.

On radiological examinations, peristalsis appears normal in the part of the esophagus above the aortic arch. Still, its function is abnormal in most patients. Contractions may be smaller in number, but their most important characteristic is their weakness, which means that the contractions do not close the esophageal lumen and allow a significant part of the barium to escape proximally.

The clinical features of the esophagus in scleroderma are heartburn and dysphagia, the former as a consequence of pronounced gastroesophageal reflux due to the incompetent sphincter and dysphagia as a result of motor impairment.

Pepsin: The Real Culprit Behind Heartburn

Pepsin is a powerful enzyme present in gastric juice that aids in the digestion of proteins we consume. It is actually an endopeptidase whose main objective is to break down food proteins into smaller parts known as peptides; the peptides are absorbed in the intestine and degraded by the pancreatic enzymes.

Although pepsin was isolated for the first time in history in the year 1836 by Theodor Schwann, a German physiologist, it was not until 93 years later that the American biochemist John Howard Northrop, part of the Rockefeller Institute for Medical Research, reported pepsin's actual crystallization and many of its functions, which would make him receive the Nobel Prize in Chemistry several years after the discoveries.

The Pepsin enzyme does not exist only in human bodies. It can also be produced in the stomach of a lot of animals in the world and starts acting in the early stages of life, collaborating in the digestion of proteins from dairy products, meats, eggs, and grains, mainly.

. The main cells of the body's stomach start with the production of a substance named pepsinogen. This proenzyme or zymogen is normally hydrolyzed and activated by our gastric acids. We lose 44 amino acids in the whole process. Ultimately, the pepsin enzyme normally contains 327 amino acid residues in its active form. All of them perform their functions at a gastric level. The loss of the 44 amino acids we have been talking about usually leaves the same number of free acid residues. This is why that pepsin works best in very low pH media.

How does it work under normal conditions?

The principal function of the pepsin enzyme refers to the digestion of proteins. Therefore, pepsin activity is usually higher in highly acidic environments meaning a pH between 1.5 and 2. The pepsin also works best in temperatures that can vary between 37 and 42 °C.

Only a small part of the proteins that reach the stomach are degraded by this enzyme, conforming approximately 20%, creating small peptides.

The activity of pepsin normally focuses on the hydrophobic N-terminal bonds that are present in aromatic amino acids. We can name here tryptophan, phenylalanine, and tyrosine, which we can find in a lot of proteins in the food we consume.

A very important function of pepsin that some authors have described takes place in our blood. Even when this claim can be controversial, it appears that tiny amounts of pepsin are present in the bloodstream, where the enzyme acts on large and partially hydrolyzed proteins that were absorbed by the small intestine right before they were totally digested.

How do we produce it?

Pepsinogen, a substance secreted by the most important cells in our stomach, also known as zymogen cells, is the creator of the Pepsin enzyme.

The proenzyme mentioned before is released due to the impulses from the vagus nerve and the hormonal secretion of gastrin and secretin, which are normally stimulated after consuming food.

When it is in the stomach, the pepsinogen mixes with hydrochloric acid, which was released by the same stimuli, fastly interacting with each other to produce the pepsin enzyme.

The pepsin is carried right after the cleavage of a 44 amino acid fragment from the original structure of pepsinogen through a compounded autocatalytic procedure.

Once active, the pepsin is able to continue stimulating all the production and release even more pepsinogen. That moment is a great example of what it is called positive enzyme feedback.

In addition to pepsin itself, components like histamine and especially acetylcholine can also stimulate peptic cells in order to synthesize and liberate new pepsinogen.

Where does it operate?

Its main place of action is our stomach. This moment can be easily explained by understanding that heartburn is the perfect condition for its execution (pH 1.5-2.5). Actually, when the food bolus is transported from the stomach to the duodenum, the pepsin enzyme is immediately inactivated if it faces an intestinal environment with a basic pH.

Pepsin also works in our body's blood. Even when this effect has already been said to be controversial among the scientific community, some researchers claim that pepsin passes into the blood, where it continues to digest certain long-chain peptides or those that have not been completely degraded.

When pepsin is no longer in the stomach and finds itself in an environment with neutral or basic pH, its function simply stops. Anyway, as it is not hydrolyzed, it can be activated one more time if the environment is reacidified.

This feature is essential to understanding some of the negative effects of pepsin, which are discussed below.

Pepsin and Reflux

The frequent return of the pepsin enzyme into our esophagus may be the origin of the damage received by acid reflux. Thus, even when the other substances involved in the production of gastric juice are also involved in this disease, pepsin is to be blamed for being the most harmful of substances.

Pepsin and other acids in reflux can provoke esophagitis, which is the initial damage but affects a lot of other systems in the body.

Important consequences of pepsin activity on certain issues may include laryngitis, pneumonitis, chronic hoarseness, persistent cough, laryngospasm, and laryngeal cancer.

Asthma caused by pulmonary microaspiration of gastric contents has also been studied in recent years. Pepsin enzyme can have an irritating effect on the bronchial tree and favor the constriction of the airway, triggering the typical symptoms of this disease: respiratory distress, cough, wheezing, and cyanosis.

Not everything is bad

Despite all the above, pepsin can also be very useful when it comes to the medical field. Also, the presence of pepsin in the saliva is an important resource to use as a diagnostic indicator for acid reflux.

In fact, there is a quick test available on the market named PepTest; this detects the presence of pepsin in the saliva and helps doctors in the diagnosis of

acid reflux.

In addition, pepsin is used in the leather industry and classic photography and in the production of cheeses, cereals, snacks, flavored drinks, predigested proteins, and even chewing gums.

Hidding from the spotlight: Hydrochloric acid

What is acidic and what is alkaline

To understand the concepts of acidity and alkalinity, we first need to understand what the pH or potential of hydrogen is? It is a value used in order to measure the alkalinity (base) or acidity of a certain substance, indicating the percentage of hydrogen found in it, measuring the number of acid ions (H +).

The pH scale normally ranges from 0 to 14, so that 7 is considered a neutral pH value, less than 7 becomes more acidic, above 7 it becomes more alkaline.

The body's acidity or alkalinity (base) can be measured by blood, urine, or saliva. The ideal pH level in the blood should range between 7.35 and 7.45, but air pollution, bad eating habits, or stress acidify the body and alter this pH; the blood reacts and steals the nutrients it needs from the rest of the vital organs to compensate for the imbalance.

In this sense, nutrition is a vital factor in achieving the optimal state of acid-base balance since there are nutrients with the ability to acidify and others with the ability to alkalize (basify).

Foods are classified according to the effect they have on the body after digestion and not according to the pH they have on their own; thus, the taste is not an indicator of the pH that can be generated within the body, as is the case with citrus fruits, which despite tasting acidic, has a completely alkaline (basic) effect on the body.

Minerals like potassium, calcium, sodium, and magnesium form alkaline (basic) reactions in the body and are found primarily in fruits and vegetables. On the contrary, foods that contain iron, sulfur, and phosphorus, such as meats, eggs, dairy products, and nuts, are acidity promoters.

Your diet should be made up of 20 to 25% acidic foods and 75 to 80% alkaline foods in an ideal world. Only in this way can we gradually create a balanced environment within the body so that it is protected from diseases and cellular deterioration.

The consequences of an acidic pH are:

- Decreased activity of the immune system
- Encourages calcification of blood vessels
- Loss of bone mass and muscle massMuscleloss
- Chronic fatigue
- pain and spasms
- Hair and deterioration of nails
- Irritated skin
- Generalized fatigue

Food Acids and alkalis are responsible for metabolic processes and, at the same time, are necessary as defense mechanisms to avoid diseases. Therefore, to have good health, it is essential to maintain a balance in the consumption of both.

About Hydrochloric acid

The stomach creates gastric acids to break down food. These acids, also called gastric juices, are very strong acids present in our stomach. Its objective is to promote the digestion of proteins that come from the products we eat.

They are composed mainly of hydrochloric acid but, in addition, they are composed of more than acids in a mixture of:

- Water

- Electrolytes (sodium, potassium, and calcium)

- Enzymes, which destroy proteins and accelerate the digestion process

One of The main components of these gastric juices, as we have already mentioned, is hydrochloric acid. Eating food triggers a set of mechanisms to facilitate digestion. First, the body releases hormones that stimulate the acid-producing cells of the stomach. These cells combine hydrogen atoms with chlorine - which we find in salt - to produce hydrochloric acid.

Hydrochloric acid is a water-based solution of hydrogen chloride gas. It is also the main component of gastric acid, an acid produced naturally in the human stomach to help digest food, as we have already mentioned. Hydrochloric acid is also produced synthetically for a variety of industrial and commercial applications. It can be obtained through various manufacturing processes, such as dissolving hydrogen chloride gas in water.

This particular acid has the ability to completely corrode a piece of metal and kill any living cell. As a curiosity to note, it must be said that the corrosive power of hydrochloric acid is a thousand times higher than that of saliva. The amount that the stomach can contain this substance is 1 to 4%.

Let's see what the principal functions of this Hydrochloric Acid that our stomach secretes during digestion

● are:

●

● It processes and digests the proteins that reach the stomach, turning them into smaller and more recognizable molecules for the Small Intestine to be more easily digested and absorbed.

● It is an antibacterial protection mechanism; that is, it is responsible for eradicating the greatest number of microorganisms that reach the stomach through what we eat. Therefore, it kills harmful bacteria and yeast.

● It is vital for the absorption of certain micronutrients, such as Calcium, Magnesium, Zinc, Copper, Iron, Selenium, Boron, etc.

● It is essential for the stomach to empty properly and to discharge the contents to the Small Intestine.

Why does it not negatively affect our digestive system?

Two to three liters of gastric juice are created a day in the stomach of an adult. Acidity and acid composition are not constant but change with flow rate. So it does not cause any damage to the stomach as long as you do not have an acid overdose.

As if the previous were not enough, there is a mucosa that lines the inner side of the stomach. This mucosa lubricates the ingested food so that it circulates more easily through our digestive system and makes an internal wall a barrier to precisely prevent it from being ingested. Finally, to ensure good digestion without problems, the stomach makes its own antacid, secreting bicarbonate to neutralize it.

As a curiosity, while food is being digested and important nutrients are absorbed, the stomach can double in size, with a capacity of 3 liters, instead of 1.5, which is its original state.

This process of digesting food can take three to four hours in the stomach. Then it passes to the small intestine, where the process can last from 6 to 20 hours until the excess nutrients are eliminated.

Effect of hydrochloric acid on pepsin

The transformation of carbohydrates has begun in the mouth with the action of ptyalin present in saliva. Chewing performs a mechanical transformation that, in addition to breaking food into smaller pieces, mixes them with saliva. This is why it is so essential to chew well. Once we have chewed and mixed the food with saliva, it passes into the esophagus and reaches the stomach. The stomach is a magnificent organ prepared to withstand very low and acidic pH levels, much like the presence of hydrochloric acid in gastric juice creates it.

The pepsin secreted in the stomach acts on the proteins. Still, for this, it needs a certain level of acidity that generates the presence of hydrochloric acid. In other words, without sufficient hydrochloric acid, the proteins will pass into the small intestine without having been sufficiently transformed, so they can cause putrefaction. On the other hand, carbohydrates that are not properly modified also continue their transit to the intestine with a greater probability of fermentation.

The importance of the acidity of hydrochloric acid

The stomach's high acidity also acts as a barrier against infection since it eliminates most of the bacteria. Acid secretion is stimulated by nerve impulses that reach the stomach, gastrin (a hormone secreted by the stomach), and histamine (another substance released in the stomach).

Fermentation and putrefaction due to inadequate digestion of proteins and carbohydrates generate bloating, intestinal rhythm problems, internal intoxication, hepatobiliary overload.

As in a chain of reactions, gastric juices support the initiation of the release of bile from the gallbladder that will act on lipids and perform its antiseptic actions. Without sufficient bile or adequate release of bile, there is physiologically more likelihood of gallstones and hepatobiliary damage in general. On the other hand, the pancreas is not stimulated. The pancreatic juices are insufficient; the pancreatic amylase cannot act properly on carbohydrates. Finally, pancreatic juice and bile association is not adequate: lipids cannot be well digested.

We could summarize by saying that when the first essential link in the digestive chain, hydrochloric acid, fails or is insufficient, the rest can fail. The basic nutrients remain without being extracted from food, in addition, certain vitamins cannot be created, such as B12, minerals such as iron, calcium, zinc or magnesium, etc. are not well assimilated.

Low levels of hydrochloric acid cause food to be digested incorrectly and increase intra-abdominal pressure. The increase in intra-abdominal pressure causes the Lower Esophageal Sphincter or Valve to open and close when it should not, resulting in the presence of reflux.

Consequences beyond the obvious

People with gastroesophageal reflux are exposed to various complications: esophagitis, Barret's esophagus, esophagitis stricture, esophageal ulcer, or gastrointestinal bleeding.

Esophagitis

It is a complication that occurs when the normal defenses of the esophagus mucosa are unable to counteract the effect of the damage produced by the refluxing acid so that the mucosa is altered. According to the intensity of the lesions produced, the following can be distinguished:

- Mild esophagitis: apparently, the mucosa is normal but microscopic damage has occurred due to the infiltration of inflammatory cells in the mucosa.

- Erosive esophagitis: damage to the mucosa is seen, and there is redness, friability, superficial ulcers, and so on.

Barrett's esophagus

The set of cells that line the esophagus on the inside is called the epithelium. The epithelium of the esophagus is different from the epithelium of the stomach. Still, when there is reflux, the epithelium of the esophagus changes and becomes the epithelium of the stomach to better support the acidity of the gastric contents at that level. This process of exchanging one epithelium for another is called metaplasia. Barrett's esophagus consists of the replacement of the normal squamous epithelium of the esophagus by metaplastic columnar epithelium and is probably due to a sustained injury/regeneration process.

To diagnose it, endoscopy (visualization of the esophagus) is used together with taking samples (biopsy) to analyze them under the microscope.

The importance of Barrett's esophagus lies in its premalignant nature. The risk of developing esophageal cancer is estimated to be 50 times higher in these patients. This is due to the following sequence of changes: metaplasia → dysplasia → cancer. For this reason, all patients with Barrett's esophagus must be followed up with periodic endoscopies; every 12 months if there is low-grade dysplasia, and every 24 months if there is no dysplasia.

Treatment for Barrett's esophagus without dysplasia will be the treatment for reflux. Treatment for Barrett's esophagus with severe dysplasia will be surgery (removal of the affected area).

Esophagitis stricture

Occurs when gastroesophageal reflux is severe and prolonged and occurs in about 10% of patients with untreated esophagitis. It is due to inflammation and fibrosis produced at this level as a consequence of reflux. It usually manifests as difficulty swallowing (especially when swallowing solid foods) and is treated by dilations.

It is advisable to take samples to analyze in the laboratory and rule out that they are due to a malignant process.

Esophageal ulcer

It is a relatively common complication of reflux esophagitis. It is more common if there is Barrett's esophagus, and they can become deep, causing even acute bleeding and perforation.

They are diagnosed by endoscopy, and a sample must also be taken to rule out that they establish a malignant process.

Gastrointestinal bleeding

It is also a common complication that should be suspected, especially when the patient has anemia due to chronic blood loss. However, massive bleeding from the mouth is rare.

Esophageal cancer

Esophageal cancer is a type of cancer that happens in the esophagus. This long, hollow tube goes from the throat to the stomach. The esophagus helps move the food you eat from the back of your throat to your stomach to digest. Cancer of the esophagus usually begins in the cells that line the inside of it. It can occur anywhere in the esophagus. Cancer of the esophagus is more common in men than in women. Cancer of the esophagus is the sixth most common cause of cancer deaths worldwide. Incidence rates vary in different geographic locations. In some regions, the higher rates of esophageal cancer can be attributed to tobacco and alcohol use or to certain nutritional habits and obesity.

Types of esophageal cancer

Cancer is classified according to the type of cells involved. Knowing the type of esophageal cancer you have helps you determine your treatment options. The types of esophageal cancer include the following.

Adenocarcinoma

Adenocarcinoma begins in the cells of the mucus-secreting glands of the esophagus. It can occur most often in the lower esophagus. Adenocarcinoma is the most common form of esophageal cancer in the United States, affecting primarily white men.

Squamous cell carcinoma

Squamous cells, which are thin, flat cells that line the surface of the esophagus, participate in this type of cancer (also called "squamous carcinoma"). Squamous cell carcinoma most commonly occurs in the upper and middle esophagus. It is the most common esophageal cancer in the world.

Other rare types

Some rare forms of esophageal cancer include small cell carcinoma, sarcoma, lymphoma, melanoma, and choriocarcinoma.

Chronic cough

The pharynx, larynx, and bronchi are the most affected; patients frequently report chronic cough (of months of evolution) that is caused by inflammation of the larynx and pharynx, as well as hoarseness (dysphonia), even bronchospasm, causing a sensation of respiratory distress (dyspnea) possibly due to the passage of refluxed material into the airways.

It is one of the causes of chronic cough that is difficult to manage since it can appear as the only symptom of reflux. Many times patients are energetically treated with drugs that act only in the respiratory tract without achieving improvement of the symptoms by not treating the cause base that is reflux.

TOOLS AND SOLUTIONS FOR A COMMON BAD

Medicines for quick relief

The best way to combat reflux is through substantial changes in diet and lifestyle. However, it is very common to find over-the-counter drugs that help relieve symptoms caused by reflux.

You can buy many medicaments for acid reflux without a prescription. However, if the affected person has symptoms that do not disappear, they should consult with the doctor.

All acid reflux medications work differently. Therefore, a combination of acid reflux disease medications may be necessary to control the annoying symptoms.

Antacids

Doctors commonly recommend antacids as a first step to relieve heartburn and other mild symptoms of acid reflux. Antacids include over-the-counter medications made primarily of simethicone.

Simethicone is used to treat symptoms of flatulence (gas) such as pain or discomfort caused by pressure, feeling full, and abdominal bloating. Simethicone comes as a regular, chewable tablet, capsule, and liquid solution that must be taken by an oral via. It is normally taken 4 times a day, after meals and at bedtime. Follow the directions on the medicine label carefully and ask your doctor or pharmacist anything you don't understand. Then, use the medicine exactly as prescribed. Do not use a different dose than the prescribed dose or more often than prescribed by your doctor.

Antacids may have some side effects, such as diarrhea and constipation, although it is something rare.

H2 blockers

H2 blockers can decrease acid production. They provide short-term relief for many people with symptoms of acid reflux. They can also help to heal the esophagus, but they are not as good as other medications. Anyone can buy H2 blockers over the counter, or the doctor can prescribe them. Types of H2 blockers include:

- cimetidine
- famotidine
- nizatidine
- ranitidine

If a person has heartburn after eating, the doctor may recommend taking an antacid and H2 blocker. The antacid helps to neutralize the gastric acid, and the H2 blocker prevents the stomach from making acid. By the moment the antacid has stopped working, the H2 blocker has already stopped the acid.

Proton pump inhibitors

Proton pump inhibitors have the capacity to minimize the amount of acid the stomach creates. These kinds of medicines are better at treating acid reflux symptoms than H2 blockers. Inhibitors can also heal the esophageal lining in most people with GERD. Therefore, doctors commonly prescribe proton pump inhibitors to treat long-term gastroesophageal reflux disease.

However, studies show that persons who take proton pump inhibitors for a long time or in high doses are more likely to fracture their hips, wrist, and spine. In addition, the patient must take these medications on an empty stomach in order for their stomach acid to make them work.

There are several types of proton pump inhibitors available with a prescription, including:

- esomeprazole
- lansoprazole
- omeprazole
- pantoprazole
- rabeprazole

The patient should consult with the doctor about taking omeprazole or low strength lansoprazole, which are sold without a prescription.

Prokinetics

Prokinetics help the stomach empty faster. Prokinetics that require a prescription include:

- bethanechol
- metoclopramide

Both medications have side effects, such as:

- nausea
- diarrhea
- fatigue or tiredness
- depression
- anxiety
- delayed or abnormal physical movement

Prokinetics can provoke problems if mixed with other medications, so the patient should inform the doctor about all the medicines you are taking.

Antibiotics

Antibiotics, including erythromycin, can aid the stomach to be empty faster. Erythromycin has fewer side effects than prokinetics; however, it can cause diarrhea.

Alternative treatments: your best allies for the body and pocket

Alkaline water

Long is the list of benefits attributed to alkaline water. Surely you have seen some ads in the media or friends have recommended you consume alkaline water to extend your life, prevent osteoporosis and cardiovascular diseases, diabetes, neurodegenerative disorders, or even the most worrying from my perspective - treat cancer.

Acidity is related to cancer development and an increase in cortisol, the stress hormone, which is harmful to our health by causing overweight, cardiovascular disease, and the development of malignant tumors.

Faced with this acidic scenario, multiple investigations seek to demonstrate the benefits of promoting alkalinity in the body. It is clear that a diet rich in fruits, vegetables, and whole grains contributes to maintaining health for many reasons, including the number of minerals that, in addition to other factors, regulate pH.

Most of the good things about alkaline water are attributed to its purported oxidative stress-reducing effect. This is because the excess of hydrogen ions leaves less oxygen available for the cells and generates more acidity. At the same time, an alkaline state implies that there are fewer hydrogen ions and, therefore, more oxygen availability.

There are several types of alkaline water available commercially. We have those that are treated with an ionization process, a process that can be done with several brands of filters, and those that are naturally more alkaline as they come from the mountains and pass through the rocks that nourish them with minerals. Some brands claim to have a pH of 9. But the question is, does the recipe for a long and healthy life really lie in consuming alkaline water every day?

Although in Japan we can read a lot of publications that corroborate the benefits of alkaline water, there is no scientific study that proves 100% of its virtues in the prevention and fights against chronic degenerative diseases in the West. The only condition with which it has been possible to relate the benefit of alkaline water is gastroesophageal reflux disease. The liquid allows counteracting acidity by preventing the activation of pepsin and exerting an antagonistic effect of the acid, reducing the annoying heartburn.

In the process of alkalizing the water, a valuable compound for the treatment of gastric acidity is produced, such as magnesium hydroxide, responsible for its alkaline pH and antacid effect. This compound is used to relieve heartburn, acid indigestion, and gastric reflux. In addition to this, a strong antioxidant potential is also produced, capable of sustaining the neutralizing effect of alkaline water after ingestion.

Some particular rules about its use

- It is good to use it first thing in the morning after waking up to eliminate any pepsin that may have refluxed and lodged in the throat during the night.

- Good to use during times of fasting, well cleared from meals.

- Gargle the water and swish around the mouth to help clear the mouth and throat.

- Swallow a little to pass through the esophagus and remove any particles inside.

Alkaline Water Precautions

- Do not overly alkalize the water. It can be as harmful as acid and can damage teeth and skin.

- Do not use alkaline water ½ hour before a meal or 3 hours after a meal. It can strongly interfere with digestion.

Food supplements

Although it is essential to consult a specialist if you have acid reflux, following a balanced diet that provides vitamins can help you combat it. The main function of vitamins is the proper functioning of the human body. However, it also helps in conditions that would not be expected, such as gastroesophageal reflux.

Although they are not part of the cure or treatment, they do play an important role in the symptoms of reflux, even more so with proper nutrition. According to studies, there is scientific evidence of the direct effects of some vitamins since they optimize any treatment. Therefore, with prior medical approval, we tell you which are the best vitamins to alleviate this problem.

Vitamin B

According to a study carried out in 2006 by the specialist Ricardo de Souza Pereira, vitamin B could help you relieve acid reflux.

The researchers involved here divided the participants into two groups, and one of them took a supplement that contained the following:

- Vitamin B6.
- L-Tryptophan.
- Methionine
- Vitamin B9 (folic acid)
- Betaine.
- B12 vitamin.
- Melatonin

Instead, people in the opposite group took treatment with omeprazole, one of the most popular for treating acid reflux.

The first group reported that several of their symptoms faded after about 40 days. This means that 100% of the people who took the vitamin B supplement experienced relief without any adverse side effects.

On the other hand, only 65% of people on omeprazole improved during the same period.

Vitamins A, C, and E

Research endorsed by several Croatian universities in 2012 evaluated the effects of antioxidant vitamins in gastroesophageal reflux diseases, Barrett's esophagus, and esophageal tumors.

The results showed that those who consumed vitamins A, C, and E through fruits, vegetables, and vitamin supplements were able to reduce the effects produced by complications of gastroesophageal reflux.

For this reason, if you consume more fruits and vegetables and supplements containing vitamins A, C and E, you will experience considerable relief. Of course, your quality of life will also improve.

Vitamin D

The main source of vitamin D is the body's own production. First, in the skin, and thanks to the ultraviolet B rays of sunlight, a precursor substance called 7-dehydrocholecalciferol, is transformed into cholecalciferol or vitamin D3. Then, vitamin D3 undergoes a couple more transformations in the liver and kidneys before it becomes active vitamin D.

Vitamin D is an important hormone that performs relevant functions in bone metabolism, autoimmunity, and cell differentiation. One of its main actions is at the intestine level, where it makes possible the absorption of the calcium ion.

Magnesium and potassium

Magnesium is a nutrient with a structure similar to that of Calcium, essential for the functioning of several important enzymatic and metabolic processes, the internal regulation of which is carried out by the kidney.

Aluminum hydroxide and magnesium hydroxide are antacids used together to relieve heartburn (heartburn or heat), acid indigestion, and stomach pain. They can also be used to treat symptoms in patients with peptic ulcer, gastritis, esophagitis, hiatal hernia, or too much acid in the stomach (gastric hyperacidity). Aluminum hydroxide and magnesium hydroxide combine with stomach acid to neutralize it. Both are available without a prescription.

On the other hand, potassium is an alkalizing mineral that helps reduce acidity due to its high pH. In addition, it is a fruit that contains a chemical that stimulates the production of the stomach lining, protecting it from the excess acid that we ingest throughout the day.

DGL

Disinfected Licorice (DGL) is a licorice extract in which glycyrrhizin, the constituent that stimulates the adrenal glands and can cause an increase in blood pressure, has been removed. DGL is widely used to support treatments for Gastritis and Peptic Ulcer Disease. In addition, due to its beneficial effects on the mucous membranes of the digestive tract, DGL is also believed to be helpful in treating acid reflux.

D-Limonene

D-Limonene is a natural substance that is extracted from citrus fruits, with a smell and taste reminiscent of freshly squeezed lemon. It has beneficial properties for the body, so it counteracts anxiety, stress, depression, stimulates the immune system, ulcers, and gastric reflux.

It is rich in vitamin C, favoring the absorption of iron. It is one of the best cleansing remedies, helping to improve digestion and relieve heartburn. It is advisable to include limonene in your daily diet due to its ability to block gastric juices' acidity and help intestinal juice.

Melatonin (or 5-htp, the precursor melatonin)

Melatonin has known inhibitory activities on gastric acid secretion and nitric oxide biosynthesis. Nitric oxide plays an important role in transient relaxation of the lower esophageal sphincter, an important reflux mechanism in patients with reflux. Other bio compounds in the formula show anti-inflammatory and analgesic effects.

Activated carbon

Natural carbon is a basic substance (together with hydrogen, oxygen, and nitrogen, it is part of all living beings and their derivatives). It is porous, which gives it the power to trap any furtive molecule in its environment. Activated charcoal helps filter undigested toxins and medications, promoting a healthy digestive system.

Black raspberries

People with chronic irritation of the esophagus from stomach acid reflux, a problem called Barrett's syndrome, would improve if they ate black raspberries, according to a study presented at the 6th Annual International Conference on Frontiers in Cancer Prevention.

Previous studies have shown that incorporating black raspberries, which have antioxidant properties, inhibits our diet's appearance of chemically induced oral, esophageal, and colon cancer. In addition, this fruit reduces DNA damage and controls the growth of tumor cells and indicators of oxidative stress.

Alkaline diet

Many of the physical ailments that we sometimes suffer, such as reflux, in our daily lives can be caused by heartburn. A good alternative to avoid these discomforts is the introduction of an alkaline diet in our diet.

As its name suggests, this diet is based on the consumption of alkaline foods, which are those that have a low acid content and increase the pH of our body. It is characterized by the substitution of processed foods, red meat, and sugars for, mainly, fresh vegetables, fruits, and legumes.

This distinction of foods is based on the pH level of foods, which is the indicator of the acid content they have. For example, alkaline foods are those that have pH levels above 7, and those below this figure are considered acidic.

However, foods considered "acidic" should not be completely eliminated, as they balance the pH level of the blood and have an important role in metabolism.

Follow the following nutritional recommendations:

- Vegetables: Consume them steamed, avoiding frying. Do not consume tomato and its derivatives (puree, sauce, ketchup).

- Fruits: Avoid acidic fruits, such as pineapple or grapes. Avoid juices made from the fruits mentioned above.

- Meats: Eat low-fat meat, skinless chicken, fish, and turkey. Avoid fatty meat, canned meats (ham, bacon, cold cuts, etc.).

- Fats: Avoid fats in general, both animal and vegetable.

- Drinks: Avoid alcohol, coffee, chocolate, tea, and carbonated drinks. You can consume decaffeinated beverages.

Avoid peppermint tea and other foods that contain this product.

● Soups: Eat low-fat soups. Avoid soups that have milk or cream.

● Bread: Avoid bread that includes whole milk among its ingredients.

● Condiments: Avoid garlic, onions, vinegar, and peppers of all kinds.

Food can also help calm inflammation of the digestive mucosa, which improves symptoms. A comparative study carried out by Dr. Vanana Panda in Bombay and published in the journal *Complementary Therapies in Medicine* compared the efficacy of some of these alkalizing foods with bicarbonate or antacid drugs. The results were that these 10 foods are excellent to counteract acidity:

1. Cucumber: Add cucumber to your green smoothies for a digestive effect similar to that of bicarbonate. Also, include it in your salads or eat two slices every so often to relieve symptoms. Cucumber contains plenty of water, which relieves acidity but also enzymes called proteases that facilitate digestion.
2. Broccoli: Broccoli is a natural antacid. That effect is the most prominent among several foods analyzed at the Kundnani College of Pharmacy in Bombay. Include it frequently in your menus, better steamed or lightly boiled, and without overdoing it with the dressing.
3. Radishes: Although it is somewhat spicy, radish is also alkaline and is among the best foods to prevent gastric reflux. It also helps the proper functioning of the liver and gallbladder. You can consume radishes as a snack and appetizer or include them

in your salads.

4. Banana: Banana is one of the foods that has proven its ability to reduce heartburn thanks to its alkalinity. Take it ripe to ensure the effect.

5. Oat milk: The mucilages in oat milk act as stomach protectors. In addition to taking the vegetable drink, you can take the oats in other forms, flakes, or grains. You can boil it in soups or leave it to soak, in water or oat milk, and add a few pieces of banana or apple.

6. Chinese cabbage: Chinese cabbage or bok choi is rich in choline, an amino acid with anti-inflammatory properties that benefits the digestive system. It is also very rich in other nutrients, such as vitamins C, A, and K. It contains more than 70 compounds with antioxidant properties, which help prevent cancer and other diseases. You can sauté it with a little boiling water in a pan for about 5 minutes.

7. Peas: peas are rich in insoluble fiber that are beneficial intestinal bacteria, essential for digestion and the assimilation of nutrients. In addition, fresh ones are so sweet because they contain simple sugars that are transformed into starch over time. Straight from the pod to your mouth, fresh and raw, peas provide abundant vitamins (folic acid and vitamin C) and minerals (iron, phosphorus, magnesium, and zinc), which would be partly lost during cooking in water. They contain abundant vitamin B1, a nutrient that promotes tranquility, delays aging, and prevents fatigue and depression. A serving of 100 g of fresh peas provides almost 20% of the vitamin B1 you need per day. They help control cholesterol thanks to beta-sitosterol and other phytosterols that reduce intestinal absorption.

8. Papaya: Papaya contains papain, an enzyme that promotes the good digestion of proteins. Because it is also high in fiber and

water, papaya is laxative and detoxifying. Half a papaya (about 150 g) meets the needs of vitamin C, 70% of vitamin A, 30% of folic acid, and 11% of vitamin E. Few foods have such doses. Most of the papayas that we find in the market come from Brazil, but if you can, choose papaya from the Canary Islands; its consumption is more sustainable.

9. Miso: Miso helps you digest thanks to microorganisms that have been shown to relieve digestive discomfort, including inflammatory bowel disease. Miso is a paste that results from the fermentation of soybeans and the Aspergillus oryzae fungus. This paste is used to make sauces and soups or to season vegetables, always using it instead of salt. It is also nutritious because it contains amino acids and significant amounts of manganese, copper, and zinc, essential minerals with antiviral properties. As it contains probiotics, you have to add them to recipes cold or when they have warmed up. 10 g of miso per person is sufficient.

10. Chamomile: Chamomile is one of the most digestive plants. Helps prevent gas from accumulating in the stomach and relieves abdominal heaviness. In addition, its smooth and pleasant flavor is ideal to finish any meal. The properties of chamomile are due to its content in bisabolol and other terpenes present in the flowers. The infusion is prepared with one or two bags of chamomile, a teaspoon of dried flowers (about 5 g), or 6 fresh flowers. In all cases, the chamomile is left in freshly boiled water for 5 minutes. You can prepare a chamomile gel or jelly by mixing the infusion with half a teaspoon of xanthan gum (for the gel) or a sheet of agar agar (for the jelly). You can use the gel as a sauce and the gelatin as a dessert. You can add a few drops of ginger juice and 2 or 3 berries to this jelly.

When consuming these foods, it is very important to try to chew them properly and at a slow pace to activate digestion processes efficiently. Likewise, it is important not to consume anything three hours before going to bed; otherwise, you will affect your body's digestion (and you will also avoid a restful sleep).

Finally, prevention is the key! A good diet can do a lot more for you than a full arsenal of drugs. Take advantage of this need to start cooking at home. In this way, you will know exactly what ingredients your food contains, since even consuming in healthy places, you can find harmful additives for your reflux problem. Likewise, commercial products such as canned, fermented, and very long-lasting foods contain highly acidic ingredients to extend their life. Fresh food will always be the best.

Choosing a different lifestyle

Complementary exercises

In addition to a good diet, exercising regularly and at a reduced intensity can help keep heartburn at bay. For example, exercises such as walking, swimming, or cycling for 30 minutes a day can help you reduce heartburn and maintain a healthy weight and stay in shape.

It is important to point out that you should not eat excessively before exercising, so a light, low-fat meal is the best option. In addition, it would be best to allow at least an hour and a half, or even two, after the meal to start physical activity.

It is advisable to drink plenty of water before exercising, as it helps digestion and prevents dehydration. Of course, during exercise, it is also very important to drink water. If you prefer isotonic drinks, better dilute them in water so that their carbohydrates do not cause acidity to appear.

What Kinds of Exercises Are Best for Reducing Heartburn?

First, aerobic exercises such as walking or swimming are more suitable. These types of exercises help improve gastrointestinal transit, reducing the risk of reflux. In addition to helping to maintain adequate weight, they also promote the control of stress and anxiety, which can be other causes of heartburn. On the contrary, anaerobic exercises, which are those that involve considerable force and high resistance, can lead to an increase in abdominal pressure, favoring the appearance of reflux.

Stationary exercises are also recommended, which are more static and without sudden movements. With them, there is less agitation of the body, and acidity is avoided. In this way, cycling is less likely to feel discomfort than if we run or jump.

Regular yoga practice helps strengthen the digestive system and ensures the proper functioning of all organs. It also helps blood circulation in the area; this means we'll have fresh oxygen and improved absorption of the nutrients we need.

Yoga is a practice that produces a sense of balance and helps to strengthen and tone muscles. At the same time, yoga relieves tension and stress. Some yoga poses do a great job of gently massaging the abdominal organs to stimulate the digestive system and also improve blood flow. Regularly practicing these yoga poses strengthens the digestive system and improves blood circulation increases oxygen supply, and better absorption of nutrients. Yoga, along with a balanced diet and lifestyle modifications, is effective in keeping gastric reflux at bay.

Finally, the risk of heartburn is also reduced if, during exercise, the trunk is kept as upright as possible. We must try not to force the part of the stomach and that the exercises we do adapt to our needs and our physical form.

Eliminating bad habits

Stop smoking

Fumar gastroesophageal sphincter relaxes the muscle that connects the esophagus and stomach and retains the first phase causing acid reflux. This muscle is in charge of keeping the food eaten in the stomach and preventing us from experiencing reflux.

It also causes inflammation of the esophagus, irritates the lining of the stomach, and increases the production of acid in it, which represents the ideal combination to suffer from heartburn.

In addition, it has been shown that tobacco and nicotine can weaken the epiglottis, a part of the larynx that stops food from passing through during swallowing and protects us from gastroesophageal reflux.

Tobacco not only damages organs that intervene in our digestion - stomach, esophageal sphincter, and sphincter-and damages higher areas of the digestive and respiratory section, increasing the risk of suffering from severe gastric disorders may increase the risk of esophageal cancer.

Reduce the consumption of alcohol and caffeine

Alcohol and caffeine cause the sphincter pressure to decrease and the sphincter to lose

strength. In particular, white wine and cava, due to their higher gas content, favor reflux to a greater extent because, in addition to reducing sphincter pressure, they favor the passage of gastric content upwards when we expel the gas.

Both of these substances can cause an increase in stomach acidity that can make reflux worse. Unfortunately, consuming decaffeinated coffee is not an option either since it has the same effect on our bodies.

Keeping stress under control

Some studies have shown that people subjected to prolonged stress situations have their heart rate and muscle tension affected and suffer from digestive problems such as reflux.

This happens because the body automatically increases blood pressure, heart rate, respiration, metabolism, and the bloodstream to the muscles in response to stress. This response is intended to help our body react quickly and effectively to high-pressure situations.

When stressful situations accumulate one after another, the body does not have time to recover. This long-term activation of the stress response system can disrupt almost every process in our body. In this matter, some of the most frequent physical responses to chronic stress affect the digestive system.

Wearing loose clothing

Wearing tight pants can cause heartburn, abdominal discomfort, and excessive gas production, among other stomach problems. Likewise, the frequent use of girdles can cause reflux, heartburn, and difficulty in proper digestion.

Don't miss out!

Visit the website below and you can sign up to receive emails whenever Malia Kōnane publishes a new book. There's no charge and no obligation.

https://books2read.com/r/B-A-MAAP-ZQSXB

BOOKS 2 READ

Connecting independent readers to independent writers.

Did you love *Complete Method For Managing Reflux Symptoms*? Then you should read *Resilience: Mastering The Art of Taking Whatever Sh*t Life Throws At You*[1] by Malia Kōnane!

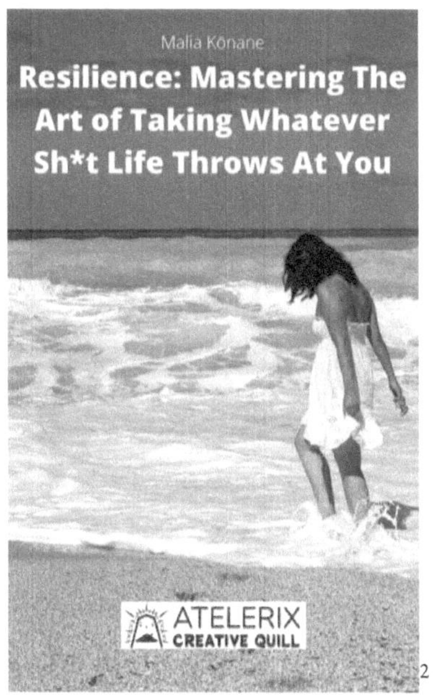

[2]

Life is a long journey that does not always follow what we had planned. On your last vacation, did everything turn out as you had planned to the millimeter? Therein lies the secret of living in the moment and knowing how to manage every contingency that arises, no matter how complicated it may seem at that moment.

Then, with perspective, are the stories that we like to tell our friends the most, "Do you remember the rebound that I got caught with the boss when he fired me and then it turns out that he did me the favor of being hooked on a better place?" And when did it seem that the plane crashed from moving so much that I ended up marrying the stewardess? " In the

1. https://books2read.com/u/4X6L5g

2. https://books2read.com/u/4X6L5g

end, it is those little moments that mark our existence, however sour they may seem at the time.

It is as painful not to reach the "Good Life" as it is terrible not to be able to imagine it. The Good Life should not be used as an illusion of occasion. It is, in any case, the ultimate goal of those who promote Scientific Socialism as the method to permanently emancipate human beings.

Under capitalism, there has been no "Good Life," even what the bourgeoisie understands by "Living Well" (according to the taste of bankers, businessmen, clergymen, and landowners) has nothing to do with a project in which, really, express the objective quality of life.

When you are done reading this book, you will have gained a lifetime of experience in just a few short hours. The stories are interesting to follow, and the challenging concepts have been made easy to understand. So get ready to broaden your horizons and adjust your expectations because you are in for one hell of a ride!

Are you ready?

If you are,

Click Buy Now With 1-Click or Buy Now to get started!

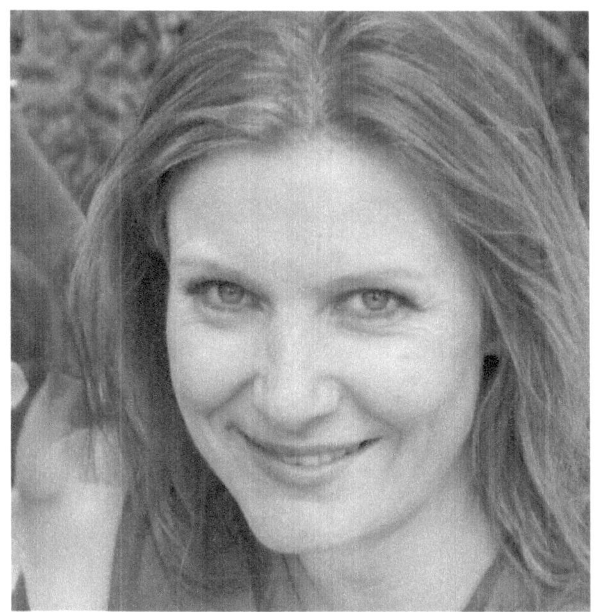

About the Author

Malia Kōnane is a 40-year-old admin assistant who enjoys meditation, playing card games, and drinking coffee. She is energetic and gentle but can also be very rude and a bit violent.

She is addicted to coffee, which her friend Sally Mason Mason pointed out when she was 18. The problem intensified in 2001. Malia has lost three jobs due to her addiction, specifically: IT technician, local activist, and clerk.

She is an American who defines herself as bisexual. She has a degree in business studies.

She grew up in a middle-class neighborhood. Having never really known her parents, she was raised in a series of foster homes.

She is currently in a relationship with Mica May Watson. Mica is 3 years older than her and works as a screenplay writer.

Malia has one child with her girlfriend, Mica: James, aged 4.

Malia's best friend is an admin assistant called Sally Mason. They are inseparable. She also hangs around with Abi O'Connor and Jayden Hill. They enjoy extreme ironing together.

About the Publisher

The love and affection created the company we have for reading and writing. Atelerix creates and publishes written works based on the knowledge and unlimited imagination of people around the world.